The ✂**Fat** [*Skinny*] American
Book One: **DIETS DECODED**

The ✂Fat [*Skinny*] American
Book One: DIETS DECODED

Annette Blake

ISBN: 978-1507859322
ISBN-10: 1507859325

✳ ✳ ✳

This book is dedicated to each and every person who is feeling hopeless and desperate about his or her weight right now.

✳✳✳
Acknowledgements

First, thank you mom and dad.

Then, thank you Jenny Craig, Dr. Atkins. Dr. Fuhrman, Weight Watchers and every other diet program and diet pill that there is for sale out there.

~ A very special thanks to Nutrisystem ~

A very personal and heartfelt thank you to those who have helped me realize that dreams do come true!

Success is only a thought away!

CONTENTS

BOOK NOTES: *In the back of the book there are a few special pages for you to take notes. You will also notice that there is a lot of blank space at the bottom of the pages of this book. That space was intentionally left blank so that the reader can write notes or scribble their thoughts.*

"When you think every diet failed, read this book. If you've ever wanted to give up trying, read this book" –Barbara, client of Annette's and advocate of her Life Success Tools and Weight Management Program.

Author Note

I've been there. I understand how you feel more than you can possibly imagine. I also know that no matter how hopeless and sad and lonely and desperate you feel, feelings *are not facts.* I promise you, change *really* is only a thought away. I'm living proof and for a long time, the "living" part was an extremely loose interpretation of what I was actually doing.

Success is only a thought away!
I promise!

-Annette

and so it begins. . .

CHAPTER 1

Change Or Die

Everyone around me (EVERYONE) constantly seems to have one thing or another to say about his or her weight. Either they are too fat or too thin or have just lost weight or they have recently gained weight…are trying to lose weight or hate their current weight…want to lose "that last" 5 pounds or need to lose [at least] 50 pounds or. . .

No matter what, it's always one thing or another when it comes to our weight (and subsequently, our eating habits). No matter where we are or whom we are with or whom we meet, if the topic of weight or eating habits comes up, we *all* have a story to tell. And in my experience, about 99% of the time anyway, the stories that I have heard are mostly delivered in some heartbreaking way and consist of tales of massive struggles and intense personal anguish. Sadly, I can't even pretend to be over exaggerating when it comes to using "massive struggles and intense personal anguish" to describe the stories I've heard. I mean this quite literally, that no one ever (well, 99% of the time, like I just said), describes their weight or eating habits with words like, 'Hey! I love my weight.' or 'Oh no. I wouldn't change a single thing about my eating habits and weight.' It's as heartbreaking to hear people's stories, as it is to know the truth about what it was that caused them to feel like they had to experience them in the first place.

Because of the high probability of you being among the elevated percentage of people who are unhappy with their weight and subsequently their eating habits, I can make the further assumption then that most of you are feeling at least a little desperate and hopeless over the *current* state that your mind and body are in. I say that because if you weren't feeling desperate and hopeless, why would you have made the decision to at least consider changing something about yourself by purchasing this book? So, if we use ourselves as the common denominator and compare ourselves to others around us, the math basically works out that most of us (un-debatably and beyond a shadow of a doubt) spend a large portion of our time unhappy with ourselves (physically as well as mentally, at least where food is concerned anyway).

Basically, there is a truth hiding within the reality of this thing that screams a very clear message to us. Unfortunately, we all pretend not to hear it. In other words, listening to people (you and me included) talk about their (our) eating habits and weight issues blatantly screams of a truth that most of us simply refuse to accept. Further, we refuse to accept it in spite of the fact that we are all smart enough to know exactly what that truth is. This truth that I'm speaking of is made up of undeniable evidence to point to the fact that we have become, *by the choices that we have been choosing to make*, a society of people who walk around behaving as though we have *no control* over our own choices when it comes to the foods that we consume.

We, in all fact and all actuality are living our lives in a state of total gluttonous food addiction yet we act like we have no idea how we got this way. Yes, I did just explicitly use the words "gluttonous" and "addiction" and like it or not, it's the truth. A very large (statistically provable) number of [fat] Americans go around living their lives and acting like they are the unwilling members of a cult run by, well, let's keep it super-sized real right from the start, the foods that we *consciously* choose to eat. The most ironic thing about this truth is that we all know it and we know it because we participated in creating it to be the truth that it is.

We plainly speak about our eating habits and food as if the food itself actually has us in a real and provable trance; like we're all participating in a massive cult overtaking led by a giant yellow clad, freakishly scary looking clown and his cohort, the king of meat patties and cheese. I mean, seriously, can we talk about this like rational, intelligent people for a little while? If not for the sake of our physical health, let's discuss it for no other reason than to gain some tangible and much needed perspective on the entire situation.

If what we've done to ourselves (at the very core definitions) isn't addiction [to food] and gluttony, what is it? I'm not saying everyone needs to rush off to a therapist or find a priest to confess to. All I'm saying is that it's time to face the reality of the situation and to stop looking at it as though we're all victims. Hopeless and desperate and obsessive and even gluttonous and addicted are all such negative words, right? Who wants to be described as any of those things? Who in their right mind *really* wants to even be negative? None of us are designed to be innately negative, so why then, do we spend so much time and use so much energy seeking more and more ways to be those things?

~ Die First, Change Later ~

As hard as it is to look backwards, it's necessary. You can't move forward without at least glancing over your shoulder to where you've just been (and in reality, still are). I would never ask you to do anything that I wouldn't and haven't already done, so I'll even volunteer to go first. But be warned. After years and years of living a life that I deemed doomed by my own personal self inflicted "suffering" and "anguish" (and sheer commitment to my own physical and emotional self destruction), I am completely incapable of being anything but brutally honest (with myself as well as all of you) about this particular subject. I've looked back and saw the truth and as hard as it was, I did it and was honest with myself about it. Therefore, I tend to tell it just how it was for me as well as try to shed some light on how it all looks from the perspective of someone who has been there, done that, shredded the triple ex men's t-shirt and never wants to go back.

That having been said, I truly believe that through suffering (self inflicted or otherwise) there is always room for growth. So here goes:

NOTE: I'm going to give you all the abridged version of my own triumphs and tribulations because like you all already know; there is always, "more to the story."

When I was a junior in college, I weighed some enigmatic, undocumented amount over 245 pounds. Before I go on, let me state for the record that I am 5'2" and mostly normal framed and can't claim to be big boned or any other adjectives that justifies me being large [obese] (gigantic is actually more like it). My best guess is that I actually weighed well over 250 pounds (probably even well over 260 pounds). The reason I can't give you a definitive weight for the time I am speaking of is because that is the time of my life where I weighed the most that I ever had (and ever will). Also, the reason I can't give you all a specific weight for that time of my life is because back then was when I had my very first *last time event*. The event of which is the motivation behind me writing this book in the first place.

I believe that we all have to have a last time event. They are events that put a pushpin in our life maps so that we have them as solid reference points (to where we don't ever want to go back to). My life map pushpin is stuck forever to the last uninterrupted morning where I woke up and weighed myself. That may not seem like a lot right now, but by the time you finish reading this book, that statement may just mean so much to you that you will recall it over and over and over. Why? Because weighing myself in the morning was something that I did obsessively. I don't mean obsessively like an anorexic or bulimic weighs themselves. I say that in spite of the fact that I probably did actually weigh myself exactly like a person with anorexia or bulimia.

I mean no offense to people of whom live their lives in accordance with those diagnoses. Truth be told though, this book is not for the psychologically diagnosed. Why? The majority of people who will identify with my story and this book have little to no use for a psychological diagnosis. Going to a therapist for our overweight and eating issues is on the bottom of the list of ways to fix those things. Therefore, we don't even consider that we are anorexic or bulimic or whatever else comes with being those things. To us, having to seek help for why we ended up the way we did means absolutely nothing to us and as you keep reading my story and this book you'll fully understand why.

So to continue, before my last time event, I weighed myself every morning (sometimes every night as well and every afternoon or randomly throughout every day and sometimes every time I was near the scale, blah, blah, blah, you get the picture). The truth for me is that each time I weighed myself, I did so hoping that one of the times that I looked down, the scale would plainly reveal to me that miraculously, every ounce of fat on my body had magically melted away, revealing my ideal and perfect weight. I'm being totally serious too so yeah, I am totally admitting to having been a tad, tiny bit delusional back then. So what though. We all have our emotionally unstable moments and it's about time we all admitted it. The reality is that this is a change or die book, not a book that is going to coddle *your* delusion and denial. If you're looking for those things, you may as well grab your receipt and bring this book right back to where you bought it and get your money back.

Now back to the morning of the event. I woke up and weighed myself before school just like I had a million times before. Only this time, when the digital display stopped at "245" it was like I heard the scale say, "Yep. Same things as the last thousand or so times you weighed yourself in the past 24 hours." I know, that seems insane and I accept that. What's hard to accept, still to this day, is what I did *next* because most of the time, I am unsure of how to portray the brevity of the situation. I mostly want to laugh my ass off about it, but there is a part of me that feels as though I should handle it more cautiously and treat it as what it really was; a total and absolute mental breakdown (of sorts).

Anyway, after the scale mocked me or at least refused to show me a weight of which I really wanted to weigh (130 skinny, perfect pounds or less) and flashed the number "245" in my face, I calmly stepped off of the scale and stood over it for a good minute and if you are anything like me, a minute is a really long time to contemplate the reality of the weight that a scale just revealed to you. If you can identify with what a really long minute of undeniable truth feels like then you'll probably be able to identify with what I'm going to say next as well. That I wish I could tell myself (and all of you) what happened inside of my mind in that very, very long minute, but I really don't remember much about it at all. What I do remember is what happened right *after* that minute. It's what happened after that that is the part that has never and will never leave my mind. Not that I want it to though because it is really a very important milestone in my life. Here's why.

After the reality of the minute passed, without a bit of hesitation, I bent over, losing my breath a little as I did because yes, even bending over took effort for me at that weight. Then I picked up the scale and calmly, yet albeit a little winded, walked to the top of my basement stairs and in a single, unplanned, uncensored, angry and vicious motion, hurled that scale down the stairs. Yes, you just read that right. I am telling you all that I got mad, no viciously angry, *at my scale* for revealing to me that I was a giant, unhealthy, fatass who weighed 245 pounds. So furious that I immediately rationalized punishing my scale by tossing it down a flight of stairs and watching it first hit the wall, then bounce against the railing, finally rolling clumsily from step to step until it landed on the cold cement floor where I was totally ok with leaving it right where it was to die a cold, damp, miserable and lonely electronic death.

You may all want to pause and take that last paragraph in before you move on. No seriously. Go ahead. I'll wait.

Good, you're all still reading which means you either identify with why I murdered my scale or at least you want to try to understand. Regardless, that means there's hope for you. Anyway, this part may suck a little for those of you who more than likely expect me to tell you that the scale incident was so emotionally dramatic for me that it became my miracle moment or *awakening* and that after it happened I woke up the very next morning and was a changed person. That the incident propelled me into a state of understanding and change and that I started eating oatmeal, wheat grass, soymilk and salads and that like being given a miracle from God Himself instantaneously lost a ton of weight (and blah,

blah, blah lived happily ever after). Right? That's sort of what you all expect, an easy solution to my (our) problem. Well…Nope. It totally did *not* happen like that for me. What *really* happened is that I woke up the next day and started to eat twice as much as I had been, which let's face it, was a lot to begin with. Fast-forward and the result of my actions led me to gain at least another 20 pounds. Probably more like 30 or 40 or who really knows how many. What also *really* happened was that I ate so much that my gal bladder and liver rebelled against me and tried to kill me and oh yeah, I developed the burden of living in a constant state of heightened and nearly deadly hypoglycemia.

Honestly though, and I'm really fast-forwarding the story now for the sake of not boring you with every, gory detail, gaining weight was just me getting *exactly* what I had been asking for. Think about it. I don't have to tell you all what I ate. It's obvious by the issues that I physically developed, but for those of you who need to read it in black and white, here's the short list: I ate and drank nothing but high fat, high sugar, overly processed, white flour enriched junk foods that have a single purpose and that was to make me fat and then ultimately kill me. Deny it if you want, but none of us need published statistics as proof that what I just said is "real" and "tangible" evidence against the foods that made up my diet.

Seriously guys and girls, keep it real ok? Nine out of ten of us are right now, as you read this, living proof that the foods I ate and that many of you still eat, are nothing more than covertly great tasting body torpedoes that once ingested, implode and systematically destroy us, one organ and body function at a time. And quite frankly, the sooner you all face it, the better your chances (of survival) will be. So liver, gall bladder and blood sugar issues (and me walking around in a constant state of sickness and emotional turmoil) were nothing more and nothing less than *exactly* what I had been calling to myself. Basically, I got exactly what I wanted. Phew. Talk about a reality check, right?

See, the thing is, the day that I tossed the scale down the stairs was not just the beginning of the end for the scale; it was the beginning of the end for my body and me too. Whomever the proverbial "they" are had some sort of subliminal affect on me because I always heard that they said that a person has to hit a personal bottom before they either die or change. In my case, not having a scale the morning after the basement stairs incident sent me into a state of utter emotional chaos. I had literally been weighing myself and holding the scale solely responsible for my weight issue(s) and eating habit(s) for so long that it became a daily neurotic and totally obsessive (but very necessary) ritual. After all, without the scale to blame, there was no one else to blame..but. . .my…..self. So imagine that next morning. Once my (scapegoat) scale was gone, what was I supposed to do? Take a look at *my* part in *my* obesity and eating habits? Seriously. Further, the last thing in the world that I cared about was my own health (otherwise I would never have gotten to two-hundred-and-forty-five-fat-and-obese-unhealthy pounds in the first place).

Therefore, being unable to stop playing the blame game, and no longer having a scale to point fingers at, I simply and quite seamlessly replaced the disappointment of waking up and not having the scale tell me that I weighed the perfect weight with eating so much food that I could just start blaming food itself for why I was fat. It was like the scale was just the middleman and once it was gone I just blamed the lead guy himself. Sadly, I am quite seriously telling it exactly like it was too. No scale. No problem. My weight became food's problem and yes, with every bite I took of every bit of food I ate, the resentment toward *it* grew until I became so helplessly entranced by food that my mind convinced me that the only way to get away from my captor (food) was to die.

And yes, I consciously felt so fat and hopeless that I really did want to die. In retrospect, if I could have died right along side of my scale, I would have. The difference between then and now is that today I know that the death that I longed for was not as much a physical one as a figurative and emotional one. Honestly, I'm not a martyr. That's why I'm still alive to tell all of you my story (and hopefully help some of you). Also, along with not being physically suicidal and thankfully physically surviving my emotional bottom, I was also blessed with years of getting to hear other people's stories (which helped *me* so much when it came time to come to terms with *my* own story).

Ultimately, telling each other our stories, before, during and after, as you all will see, keeps us all in check. That being said, I hope that you all come to learn the same lesson that I did and eventually understand what I'm about to say because it's very important. Today, after years of my own journey to acceptance, most of the time that I hear people's stories I am reminded of how I *don't* want to ever be again. It's one of the biggest reasons for me to be grateful when I am having a hard time today and it has helped me from ever having to go back to being that girl who tossed a scale down a flight of stairs as if *my* issues were *its* fault. It's also one of the biggest gifts that I could ever get from writing this book. To know in my heart that someone will use my experiences as reminders for them of how they never want to be (again) would truly let me know that none of us are alone in this thing.

~ My Story + Your Story = <u>OUR</u> Story ~

Obviously there is more to my story than I just told you. There's always more to a story, you know? From this point forward though I am choosing to focus mostly on the positive things that happened. I will touch on some really hard things that I "went through" to get where I am today but those points, as you will see, are so much less relevant than the overall end result that they are not even worth fully mentioning. All that matters from this point forward is that 1. You keep reading and 2. That you believe with all of your heart and soul that if you want to change (even one thing about your weight or eating habits), you can and *will* do it. I can actually guarantee it but you'll have to keep reading to find out more about that.

About a year after the scale tossing incident I basically lived my life in a food induced coma and trance. Therefore I only knew a few things that happened in that time period for sure. One thing I knew was that I had gained a lot of weight. I mean I knew I gained a lot of weight and weighed a ton, metaphorically speaking of course, but it did, in all reality, actually *feel* like I weighed a ton. I also knew that my health was failing. I knew those things because of something so unbelievably bizarre and apropos that it is still cathartic for me to be sharing it all with you even right now.

The reason I knew how unhealthy and fat I had gotten was because one of my classes at college was in a building without an elevator. Stop and think about that sentence for a few seconds before you read on. Maybe even read it a few times out loud. After you've done that tell yourself, no, give yourself permission to laugh a little at this point (and from this point forward as well). Why? Because the fact that I discovered how fat and unhealthy that I had let myself get was because of having a class in a building without an elevator truly, on a very fundamental and literal level, is actually very funny. Besides, finding the humor in it all may actually save your life, (like it saved mine).

No, my first thought was not, 'Oh damn. I'm fat and unhealthy and I know this because this building does not have an elevator.' That would have been too easy and a little too obvious; two things my life lacked a lot of at that point. How I did discover the truth was a little more dramatic and a lot less blatant. It was a really hot, humid, summer day and I was trying to get to class and was running a little late. My class was on the third floor of the no elevator building..........and just so you all know, I'm emotionally getting out of breath just recalling that day.

So anyway, I rounded the corner of the second floor stairwell and was so out of breath that I had to lean up against the old, Victorian era heater that was against the outside wall just under the large multiple paned stairwell windows. I knew that there was no way that I could keep going until I caught my breath so I basically had no other choice but to pull my super-sized self over for a quick break. I couldn't even realistically take another step forward until I stopped panting, which was par for the course for me. That day was no different. Not to mention the fact that my heart felt like it was literally beating out of my chest.

So there I stood, other students speeding past me in a hurry to get to class and all I could do was pant and hiss and sweat. I was basically stuck there for a few minutes until I caught my breath enough to at least begin the tedious journey up the next and final flight of stairs. Oh, I should add that there weren't even a lot of steps but to me, at that time, each step was like climbing Mt Everest. That day, in that heat and humidity may have been the longest physical journey of my entire life because once at the top of the stairs, I still had to trudge down the long hallway that led around a few sharp turns that would finally bring me, still panting, hissing and sweating, to my classroom and then finally, to my desk.

There I was, finally at my destination and for the first twenty minutes of that class I sat at my desk, partially hunched over and staring out of a window to my right while wanting to cry as I finally and totally caught my breath. Here's the thing though, at some point during that twenty minutes, some weird emotional purging type thing happened to me. This is the part that you may want to really pay attention to. . .While I was looking out of the window and catching my breath I was also stuck in a redundant thought pattern of thinking about myself climbing those stairs. I thought about the stairs and how I was panting and hissing and how I was forced to stand to the side while trying to catch my breath as the herd of able-bodied students sped by me.

Each time the story replayed in my head, another detail would pop up and whirl around in my brain triggering even more thoughts of the stairs; and not even that many of them…panting, hissing, clutching my chest to cover my visible heart beat…the beads of sweat dripping off of my snotty running nose…exhaustion setting in as I approached that top step…facing the seemingly endless hallway that led to my class…and before I knew it, I was literally smiling and ended up busting out laughing out loud. To this day I have no idea what I found so funny about that particular journey. Further, wanting to laugh and cry at the same time is well, just weird but that is exactly what I felt at that time.

Here's an important note though, I honestly hadn't laughed at anything in such a really long time that laughing at all was sort of surreal and weird for me. The laughter of that day is an important pinpoint on my life map. The thing is, I remember those moments, the wanting to laugh and cry and catching my breath fully, as if they happened in super slow motion. From the time I stood on the landing of the stairwell to the moment that I laughed (at myself) in that class are moments that are forever carved in my mind.

And that ladies and gentleman, like it or not, was and will forever be, *my awakening*. My proverbial bottom. The turning point. The life changing event that, whether I liked it or not, would become my defining moment. Nope. I didn't get a bright light moment or get woken from a sound sleep by three ghosts who refused to let me wake up until they showed me the errors of my ways. And no one extra close to me died from a food related heart attack and shook me to my core, causing me to change my ways. For me, my turning point was simple and extremely subtle and showed up in the form of laughter (at myself).

The thing is, acceptance is acceptance no matter which angle you look at it from and what I needed was a good, healthy dose of it. That's why realizing how ridiculous it was to be hissing and huffing and puffing halfway up a flight of stairs (at my young age) and then spending twenty minutes trying to catch my breath fully and being able to laugh at myself really is a great awakening moment. Not to mention (oh-my-God!), what happened next!

CHAPTER 2
Learn to Laugh. Learn to Live? It's Your Choice.

Me laughing at myself wasn't so much about the laughter itself or even the specific time and place. It's more about an actual *point in time* where my body and mind merged (after a really long time of total and utter disconnect) and sent a message out to the proverbial "they" or Higher Power or Universe or whatever entity existed outside of the psychosis of my own thoughts and behaviors and made the simple yet bold statement, "It's over." Not over as in the trials and tribulations of the thing itself. That part can't just disappear as easily as a passing thought. It took me a long, long time to get to the obese and unhealthy place where I was so getting out of that mess could not possibly happen over night.

What did happen at that moment and time where I was able to laugh (at myself, or the situation or whatever I found amusing) is that my perception of the situation instantaneously changed (dramatically and totally in spite of myself)? What I'm saying is that my life, via a single thought which was followed by a small action instantaneously changed and I abruptly and instantly went from a pathetic, self-loathing, unhealthy, seriously obese, young female to well, something other than those things. The something else part is a sort of enigmatic and vague thing itself, even to this day. What matters is that my recollection (thoughts) triggered an action (laughter) and that action triggered a change (end result). I later met someone who would explain what happened to me, in detail, and I can't wait to tell you all about that but for now, let's stick with what happened next.

No, I did not wake up the following morning and become that oatmeal and salad eating person who I already talked about in an earlier chapter. What I did wake up to was a new vision of what my life *could* be. Since I had been given a solid vision of what my life *had* been, my best guess is that I really only had two choices come the next morning. Either change, or stay the same. I guess we'll call it acceptance because I immediately knew that what I had been eating for breakfast (diet Pepsi and whatever chips or sugar laden cereal was immediately available) was probably not really doing me much good. Those are the things that I ingested every single day prior to the stair-climbing day at college. You know, the morning of the day where I huffed, puffed, hissed, panted and groaned my way up three flights of stairs and then landed at my desk and spent a good twenty minutes trying to recoup from the long, long, long, lonnnnng journey. I knew, however vague that knowledge was, that I did not want to be the hissing and panting girl anymore. I had no idea what I *did* want to be, because, let's face it, I wasn't one hundred percent sure of what was going on with me or my brain (or body) at that point, but living the life I had and looking backward was no longer even an option.

In the days and months to follow, I began pulling away from soda and drinking more water. It actually happened almost unconsciously because I never remember making the decision to quit soda. It just started happening. I also started choosing wraps and salads at the food courts at school. I ate those instead of getting into my car and driving five miles from campus to get to McDonald's where I would stuff my face with Big Macs (notice the "s" at the end) and chicken McNuggets and yes-biggie-size-my-fries please. It's probably pretty important to mention that I not only would leave school on my breaks between classes to go to McDonald's or Burger King, but I would stop at one or the other (or both) on my way home after school as well.

Those eating *events* are on the top of the list of things that stopped immediately after the stair climb day. I would love to say that I didn't go through periods where I missed fast food. The truth is that I did miss it. Sometimes I missed it a lot and wanted to rush out and get some. I later found out that the reason I craved that kind of food was that my body was literally withdrawing from it. I won't go into the details of why our bodies crave junk food, but I will say that once we cut them off from it, there is a real period of time that it takes for our bodies to readjust to *not* eating that kind of food.

There are actual scientific facts about what happens to our bodies when we cut them off from fast food. If you need to read more about it, please feel free to look it up online. My guess is that if you're anything like me though, those facts don't really matter right now. What does matter is not feeling so hopeless and upset about your current weight. Therefore, it is very important to immediately acknowledge that fast food is *not* meant to be consumed daily. Then accept that fast food, when eaten gluttonously, is (IS!) addictive. Those are two things that must be accepted right away, even if you are saying in your head that already know that. Knowing it and accepting it are two very different things.

After I accepted that fast food was not meant for daily consumption, I had to then actively change my thinking about fast food and I really mean that I did have to do it right away because drive-thru meals and convenient store foods made up almost all of my daily food intake. I literally lived on Combos and Cheese Doodles and fries and burgers and milk shakes and whatever other super-sized, super quick, super unhealthy food I could get my hands on. So I had to consciously think about eating a fast food meal from beginning to end *before I actually ate it*. I had to do the same thing for convenient store food. I did it by asking myself three life-changing questions: ***How would I feel buying it? How would I feel eating it? How would I feel after I ate it?*** Those three questions became part of my daily thinking and they still are a very important part of my life to this day.

I am going to pause briefly right now and *strongly* suggest that you write those three questions down somewhere or maybe text them to yourself or at the least bookmark this page. I am suggesting that because before you even finish this book, you'll probably be presented an opportunity to use them. A funny story about that is that my boyfriend was reading a rough copy of the manuscript for this book and the day after he started reading it, he asked me to grab him some food from Taco Bell on my way home. I did just as he asked and got him everything that he asked me to, no questions asked. The next day he came to me and very casually said, "I should have asked myself your three questions before I ate all of that Taco Bell." He spent the rest of the day with a sick stomach.

My boyfriend started using the three questions in spite of himself and it made me really happy because part of being a weight loss consultant and coach is knowing when and who not to interfere with until they come to you and ask for help. I'm not saying that my boyfriend needs my help with his food issues. It's not my place to say that or assess him and his eating habits. What I can say is that 99% of the people I know or meet has some sort of issue when it comes to, at the minimum, making good choices about the food that they eat. Also, from years of experience working with people who have added those three questions into their daily lives, even when they didn't think they could use them, I can say with absolute certainty that their lives have drastically changed because of those questions.

Hopefully you will at least write the questions down or make a note of the page they are on so you can refer to them if you need to. Especially as you continue to read this book and are faced with making decisions about foods that you rely on and know are probably not doing your mind and body much good. The three questions, once you know them, force you to be honest with yourself. If there are foods that you contemplate or feel guilty about eating or just plain make you feel awful when you eat them (because you eat too much of them), then apply the three questions to those foods and see what happens. For example, if you buy a quart of ice cream and eat it all, maybe ask yourself the three questions before you buy the next quart and see what happens. If nothing else, you may save yourself a night of going to bed feeling bloated. You may save yourself a morning after filled with shame, guilt and remorse too. You know those mornings when you wake up mad at yourself for not having the self-control to stop eating the entire bucket of ice cream or whatever your food overindulgence of choice is.

For me, there was a lot more work to be done than adopting those three questions. I also added something else into my daily life. Laughter. At first, my laughter was mostly at myself (and FYI, I don't want a single e-mail or letter telling me that laughing at myself is bad or wrong or blah, blah, blah). This is *my* path and for me, laughing at myself was and still is a cathartic act with solid routes in acceptance. Frankly, I am so grateful for it that I will defend it with the very life that it saved. Why? Because laughing at myself does not mean that I was laughing *at* myself. It simply means that I realized that the choices of which I had been making and the lifestyle of negativity and chaos and total food addiction and cult like following that I chose to embrace was not only insane, it was quite literally hilarious when placing it next to a rational, well thoughts out life filled with truth and reality.

I personally believe that we all need more laughter. For a very long time I let things like food and the scale have so much power over me that I forgot how to laugh. I was totally miserable and kept right on the track of being more and more miserable. I know now I was miserable because of the choices that I was making but back then, I had no idea. Not until that day that I laughed at myself and realized that I was where I was because of the things that *I* did. It's alright if you can't laugh at yourself yet but trust me, finding fault in the ridiculous things that we do to ourselves then finding a way to laugh about them may save your life someday. That may not make a lot of sense to you right now, but it will. I promise.

~ Satisfaction Guaranteed ~

How many times have you said, "I'll start [a diet] tomorrow" and how many Wednesdays or Fridays or whatever-days have you told yourself, "I'll start again Monday"? How many times have you stepped on the scale hoping it would tell you *any* number other than the one that you already knew it was going to tell you? Be real with yourself. How many mouthfuls of food have you chewed, swallowed, and then immediately regretted yet took another mouthful and another and another until you temporarily ate the feelings of regret away?

Right now, as you read this, you are sitting at a critical point in your own life. I know that because you never would have purchased this book if you weren't feeling desperate and hopeless and seeking help for your own food "issues" (addiction) and/or out of control weight gain. I'd tell you how proud I am of you for making the choice to at least pursue change, but we all know that someone else being proud of us when we are feeling hopeless has about as much power over propelling us into a state where we desire to change as another round of biggie fries and a milk shake has. So instead, I'm going to do something that you definitely do not expect and trust me, by the time you finish reading this chapter, any doubts or feelings of being hopeless will be completely and absolutely gone. I'm going to offer you a 100% guarantee. Yes, you read that right. You probably didn't know that this book came with a guarantee, did you? Well, it does and I refuse to make you read another page without giving all of you the one thing that you want more than anything in the entire world and that is hope.

So here goes. No matter how many times I tell you all that I know exactly how you feel, I am fully aware of the fact that for the most part, me telling you that falls upon deaf ears. The beginning of any end, just like the end itself, comes at a price and identifying with others, is, at this point, too high of a price for any of you to pay. Sure, you may, at some gut level, know that I have been where you are right now. You may even have a strong desire to want to identify with me and my story, but right now it's like the devil and angel sitting on your shoulder scenario. The angel is telling you to identify and that there is hope for you while the devil is telling you to stop reading this and rush out for another round of biggie sized drive thru with a side of family sized skittles and a milk shake. Therefore, I don't expect you to (fully) identify with my "story" (yet). I'm a realist. I didn't get where I am by not understanding all of our stories, like the exact one where the angel told me to change or die while the devil told me that a round of biggie size and a milk shake would make dying *so* worth it. That having been said there is one thing that I do expect each and every one of you to have at this point. I expect you all to at least have the desire to change.

Sure, some of you may actually have to put this book down at this point and go and grab a 6 pack of cupcakes and some chips or a burger and fries and that's ok. All I ask is that on your way to the gluttonous food indulgence, you tell yourself that nothing changes if nothing changes and that all you are doing is prolonging the inevitable. Then commit to coming back to this book ASAP and either start reading it from the beginning or start right here, where you left off. For those of you who have the desire to change and are ready to start changing immediately, keep reading and welcome to the beginning of the new you that is beyond your wildest imagination!

~ Change is Inevitable ~

Even having nothing more than the desire to change is in all actuality, at its core, change. Even the tiniest desire to change does something enormous to your thought process. The first thing it does is stops your brain from thinking that it does *not* want to change. You don't even have to understand that on a rational level to have it work for you. All you need to understand right now is that in order to change *anything* about yourself *you* actually have to participate in that change and that this step in the process is *inevitable*. Even deciding *not to change* causes change. In other words, *if* you have a *true* desire to not continue to feel fat and hopeless and defeated, *you* are going to have to be the one to actually do something about it. Don't panic. I'm here to help, but I'm a weight loss consultant and life coach. I am not a genie in a bottle of whom can grant you three wishes where you will magically be cured of your weight and food maladies. I will however do anything that I possibly can to help you. I'll start by offering you a 100% satisfaction guarantee.

It's more than likely something that no one else will ever offer you. First, understand that there is, of course one condition to the guarantee. It is sort of obvious by what I just wrote in the last chapter but in case you missed it, I can only guarantee you'll be satisfied if first *you* commit to actively and fully participate in the process. See, what I have to offer you is a set of tools that, if you use them, will *guarantee your success*. Yes, I just told you that I can give you the tools that you (all of you, no matter how hopeless or bad you think your situation is) can use to change whatever it is about yourself that has caused you to seek help for your hopeless situation. Be it your weight (obesity), or eating habits or both or _____ (fill in the blank with whatever *you* want to work on). These tools can help you *fix yourself*.

Really, my Life Success Tools are way more than I am making them out to be. For now though I just want to give you an overview because I know from my own personal experience how overwhelming all of this can be. For now, just know that these tools, once you learn how to use them (and believe me, it is easier than you all think), will help you create a life that is beyond your wildest imagination. Not just a mediocre life but also a life you always wanted and dreamed of having but always believed was out of your reach.

For now all you need is the desire to change. That's it.

Are *you* ready?

CHAPTER 3
Your BEST Life Begins Right Now!

When I start to work with people who have weight "issues" or food "issues" I always start by telling them parts of my own story. I do that because it lightens the blow (a little) and let's them know that I truly do understand where they are as well as giving them a glimpse into where they are able to go. It also eases the pain of what comes next -- the cold, hard reality of the thing that we are *all* facing, acceptance. **Acceptance** is actually the first and most important tool that you'll put into your life toolbox. It's the one tool you'll need to learn how to use before anything can change. You actually need acceptance in order to fully achieve even the *desire* to change.

It has to be that way because unless we all accept ourselves as being where we are as a result of the choices that we've made (and that we didn't get where we are by anything other than *our own free will*), we are not in the position to change anything at all. Without acceptance we are stuck in that place where we *want* to change but are unwilling to actually participate or have a true *desire* to change. Good news and bad news, change is an action word. Bad news, it works in both directions.

Your Personal Success Toolbox

* **Acceptance** *

Like I just said, the very first tool that you absolutely need to put into your toolbox is **acceptance**. It is crucial and non negotiable. It doesn't matter what your acceptance tool looks or feels like. It can be laughter, tears, anger, apathy, rage, a stop sign, a pencil. It can be a Big Mac at this point for all I care. All that matters is that *you* personally discover a thing that will <u>force you</u> to *accept* the fact that who you currently are is not who you want to continue to be. You don't have to identify why or how anything else just yet. Keep it simple. Finding a way to initially accept things should not be complicated. It isn't hard to find this tool and it can and probably will change at various times along the way so don't panic and think that you have to get a perfect and forever tool right away. What I'm saying is that right here, right now, all that you *have* to do is find something tangible that will force your mind to take an honest look at your life.

    Do you hate your weight? Do you hate your body? Do you hate the scale? Do you hate the chocolate that you know you should stop eating gluttonously yet can't? What is making you feel hopeless? What is making you continue to do the things that are self-destructive and of which are beating you up emotionally and of which you cannot stop? By identifying some of the things that are making you keep doing the same things over and over, you are in the beginning stages of accepting those things as real choices that *you* and no one else has made and continue to make. Does answering those questions make you happy or sad or angry or apathetic or _____? Start to honestly assess what it is about yourself that you don't like and then ask yourself how you feel without reacting or putting an action to the feelings. What I'm saying is to start to have honest dialog with yourself about yourself and do it without going into denial and rushing off to eat something to try to make the process stop.

    This step is very important because once you begin to accept responsibility for how you got where you are today (let's call it your current destiny), you can begin the process of changing those things so that you can start to create a whole new destiny. In other words, ask yourself the hard questions and then have enough respect for yourself to answer those questions honestly. If you have to write them down, do it.

Keep a journal or a notebook or a napkin but take the steps necessary, whatever those steps are for you, to start accepting that you are where you are because of choices that you and no one else has made.

Most of you will get those basic concepts of acceptance right away. Honestly it's only as scary and complicated as you choose to make it because there are really only two true choices when it comes to acceptance. The first is that you accept things for what they are and realize that you are responsible for how and why they got that way. The second choice is that you don't accept things for what they are and you continue to seek things outside of yourself to blame for how and why they are the way they are. Acceptance or denial. It's your choice and part of acceptance is realizing it *always* has been that way.

At the very heart of acceptance is one, unchangeable thing, honesty. At the very heart of honestly is the desire to change. At the very heart of change is where you will find the key to moving away from the old you and toward the new and changed you. It's a process that moves you away from negative thoughts and actions and results and toward positive ones. Understandably, actually working acceptance to its full capacity may take some time and it *will* take a lot of effort but the results will come to you fairly quickly. I said quickly though and not completely. So for now, let's just keep pushing onward and avoid any opportunities to let negative thoughts block the forward momentum.

* Destiny *

The second tool that you are going to be adding to your toolbox is the tool of **destiny**. Destiny is the tool that makes it so that once you accept your part in your current destiny you can learn new ways to use it to reshape your next and all future destinies. What I'm saying is that, regardless of what you have thought up until this point, you don't just have a single, fated, binding destiny that is assigned to us at birth or by God or some other pious or powerful entity. The entire fate and destiny thing is what got many of you in the house of perpetual hopelessness in the first place. That line of thinking is exactly why you have spent months and years thinking that you are actually destined to always be fat and unhealthy so why even bother to try to change it. Right? How many of you have thought that being fat and unhappy *was* your destiny so why bother to fight it?

Well I'm going to tell you that the very principal of that line of thinking is all a load of crap and none of it is true at all. Your destiny is totally and completely up to you. Being fat and eating unhealthy did not get fated upon you and you are *not* a victim to those things. Should I repeat that last sentence for you, especially the part about you not being a victim? The first tool in your toolbox is acceptance and this is a good time to grab it and use it because I'm about to give you a much needed reality check.

The absolute truth is that you are fat and unhealthy because of the choices that *you* made and the foods that *you chose to eat*. Accept it. Right here and right now. Don't try to deny it and do not allow your mind to trick you into thinking that it is anyone else's fault but your own. You are where you are and weigh exactly what you do because of you and no one else. Your weight and health are *not* the way they are because of your genes or some pill that you're taking and no, you are *not* the victim of some predisposed condition upon which you are eternally doomed to suffer from.

I have heard so many people including people I have worked with, whine and complain about how they are fat and unhealthy *because* of their thyroid or their genes or some other medical diagnosis. Many blame a pill for why their weight is out of control. They say that they gained weight because of side affects from the illness or the pill they take to help with the illness. Sure, I understand that weight gain is listed on some pills as a side affect, but what I'm saying is that a pill cannot dictate a person's destiny. Neither can a medical diagnosis.

If you are a person who has accepted your weight gain as a secondary condition to something else, such as a medial diagnosis or treatment (like a prescribed medicine), then you will also tend to be a person who believes that you are a destined victim to obesity. You are also among some of my hardest cases but I can assure you that my Life Success Tools will work with 100% accuracy *if* you first accept *your* part in your current situation. I am not saying that you do not have actual medical conditions of which actually does affect your weight. What I am saying, and I am saying it with absolute certainty, is that 90% of the time people you are using your real medical condition as an *excuse* to become and stay fat. Sadly, if you stay on the road to that destiny, you will more than likely gain a lot more weight than is normal for your diagnosed condition. In other words, having a true medical diagnosis does not give you an open invitation to hop aboard the express train to obesity. Being sick with a real illness is one thing. Using that illness to deny responsibility for your severely poor eating habits and weight gain is another thing altogether.

Part of accepting your current destiny (so you can change it) is acknowledging that most of the time the initial medical diagnosis is actually due to your poor eating habits and obesity in the first place anyway. Sadly, that is a cold hard reality that becomes a very hard thing to accept. Still, your situation is *not* hopeless. You just have a little more work to do when it comes to understanding your part in your current destiny. So if you are one of those people who have diabetes or thyroid issues or high blood pressure, let me assure you that although you do need to seek a physician's advice prior to making any drastic changes to your diet, you can start changing your *thinking* around food *right now*.

It's time to stop hiding behind any and all excuses that you've used to keep you headed in a self destructive path and straight to a destiny that has no other end but hopelessness and despair. I've worked with people who have had really difficult medical conditions to deal with and honestly, a few of them truly had almost all medical and scientific odds against them but they used my tools and lost weight and achieved success in spite of those odds. I believe that the power of positive thinking is a far more powerful force than any other force that exists.

Take a few moments to let everything from the last few paragraphs really sink in. Be confused or skeptical or even get angry if you have to. Laugh if that is what acceptance feels and looks like to you but no matter what else you do at this point, you absolutely must accept that you are where you are, right now, in your current destiny, because of the choices that *you* and no on else made. Read those last few sentences a few times if you need to. Let it sink in. really accept it. Then, since we are accepting things completely, accept that you are not stupid and that you are now and have always been aware of the ideals of "right and wrong" (however loosely interpreted you need to make those concepts, you need to use them right now) and that includes what is right and what is wrong to eat.

No, I am not asking you to accept a reality that consists of you waking up tomorrow and eating oatmeal and salads (unless those things are things that you really want to start eating). All I'm saying is to start to accept that fast food and soda and chips and chocolate and ice cream and whatever else you personally used to get to a point of hopeless obesity were all basically negative and wrong choices; that you are where you are because of you and no one else (including food so stop blaming it).

Actually, stop blaming everything and everyone else for your hopelessness. No matter how difficult it is and how much it hurts to accept things for exactly how they and how they got to be the way they are, it's time to suck it up and deal with the truth. It's time to point the finger of blame where it really belongs, right back at yourself.

Then, on the back of accepting your previous destiny, the one filled will negativity and unhealthy choices, quickly tell yourself that anything prior to right now is an old destiny and nothing more. It's the past, not the present or future. Then tell yourself that you can erase it and create a brand new destiny starting right this very second. A destiny that suits who you *really* want to be so much better than the one you had just been living. It really, really is that easy. Trust me. It's a thought and a very powerful one. All you have to do is think the positive thought then positive actions will follow and naturally and without much effort, positive results will happen. All of that is guaranteed if you keep acceptance in the mix right from the start.

First you accept things for how they are and then you accept your part in all of it. Then you gain awareness of your past destiny and through that awareness, you get to create a totally new destiny. So right now you are standing at a critical turning point. You can be all dramatic and uptight about it and have a hissy fit and run to the nearest drive-thru and try to biggie size the reality away (which I promise you, will never happen) or you can simply just grab your new tools from your brand new [life] toolbox and start to build a new, non-dramatic, non-hopeless, reality driven, happy life.

Your next destiny really is up to you! You can choose to continue to be a victim (of yourself) or choose to change and stop setting yourself up for constant failure. The thing about all of this is that it goes either way. *You* choose to accept things or not. *You* choose to move in a positive direction or not. It has always been that way. It's like the law of gravity and has no emotional attachment to you whatsoever. If *you* choose to be negative (fat) and hopeless, you will be given opportunity after opportunity to continue to be negative and hopeless. Subsequently, if *you* choose to be positive and happy, you will be given opportunity after opportunity to be positive and happy. It is now and always has been up to you.

If you need proof, think about a single time in your life when you woke up and were grumpy and unhappy about your weight. Instead of accepting that you were grumpy and unhappy about your weight and letting it stop there, what did you do next? Did you make the decision to weigh yourself anyway, even though you knew the scale would just give you another reason to be grumpy and unhappy? Maybe you went and ate something horrible for breakfast like you know, three donuts and a large coffee with eight sugars. The truth of the matter is that you woke up grumpy and unhappy, chose to deny the reality of those things and change them, therefore asking for more opportunities to stay grumpy and unhappy.

Had you chosen to accept that you woke up grumpy and unhappy then accepted it and made a conscious decision to not stay that way, your entire day would have been different. I get that maybe changing your destiny may be a tough concept to grasp right now. It almost seems too simple and I get that. It really is simple though. For those of you (who are like me), I needed a lot more convincing. That's where the next tool for your toolbox comes in really handy

* Gratitude *

Although this one tool is likely *the* most important concept you will *ever* come across (in all aspects of your life), I'm only going to explain it briefly. It isn't that I want to make light of the brevity of this particular tool. It's that we're all adults here and I believe in all of you. I believe that you will get it or at least try to get it or at the minimum have the desire to get it. Regardless, it's so important that I probably should write an entire book about it. With me though, I function on faith these days. Not a pious and Godly, religious faith but a faith in people and how strong we all really are. That's why I listen when my gut tells me that sometimes a thing is so important that if offered up to the receiver properly, the importance of it speaks for itself.

First, keep in mind that I believe in you. Maybe that doesn't matter too much to you right now so I'm going to help you to start to believe in yourself, which is something you probably haven't done in a really long time. No worries though. It's actually not that hard to do. All you have to do to begin is to start being grateful. **Gratitude** is the next tool you'll be adding to your toolbox and along with acceptance, you need to start using gratitude right away (and often). I suggest that you start when you wake up tomorrow. Before you even put your feet on the floor, be grateful. It doesn't matter what you're grateful for, just find something to be grateful and then take a moment and acknowledge it with a thought of gratitude.

Maybe you can be grateful for your comfy pillow or that you woke up when you needed to. Just find something to be grateful for.

Oh, and forget any previous life thoughts on gratitude, like the one you're telling yourself that says you've *always* been a grateful person. Then free yourself from the thought that you were raised in such or such religion and that gratitude isn't a problem for you because you went to church or believe in God. Those thoughts are lies because if you were *truly* grateful, you wouldn't be reading this book and looking for help (or feeling fat and hopeless and out of control).

At this point, you will have to have some faith in me when I tell you that the kind of gratitude that I'm asking you to have is a new kind. It is not a religious gratitude that is attached to "good vs. evil" and the old argument of right and wrong. This gratitude is personal to you and the new destiny that you are creating. It's a game changing gratitude that isn't tainted by the old religious concepts of right or wrong and no one else gets to assign a meaning to it for you. It's part of the guarantee that I told you about. It's a gratitude that can and will free you from anything negative (including your old self).

To begin to understand this kind of gratitude and to start using it to build some over needed belief in yourself, all you have to do is start being grateful. Just start by practicing being grateful for anything. The sun or the clouds or maybe the bowl of cereal you're going to eat. Be grateful that you woke up or that you have a bed to sleep in. Be grateful for your slippers or your job or go out on a limb and be grateful for every bite of food that you have ever eaten, even the ones that got you to a point of hopelessness and despair (or even suicidal thoughts or actions). Why?

The answer is simple and I wish I could claim it as my own, but it isn't mine at all. It was something that was given to me when I was at my lowest point. Therefore, I am so grateful for it that I feel that in order to continue to be blessed with having it work for me, I need to pass it on to you. Therefore, I am merely paying it forward in hopes that it helps you like it helped me. The reason that being grateful is so important is because the act of being grateful triggers a bunch of other thoughts inside of your brain that become like little negative-thought land mines. Simply put, if you are being grateful (for anything), negative thoughts instantly have no other option than to start to disappear.

This is why:

Negative thoughts lead to → Negative actions, which lead to →
Negative Results
 Positive thoughts lead to → Positive actions, which lead to →
Positive Results

If you are thinking (any negative feeling) and continue to allow being (any negative feeling) to rule your thoughts, then those thoughts *will* lead you to engage in (any negative) actions. Those (negative driven) actions with lead to (negative driven) results. Once the forward momentum is going toward being negative, it will just keep right on going in that direction *unless you choose to stop it.* Gratitude is *the* most powerful weapon you can use against negativity.

If you think about it realistically, then you will start to understand why you ended up exactly where you are right now. For a very long time you have been waking up in a state of absolute [self inflicted] despair and hopelessness and now you know it's your own fault. Your first thoughts of the day have mainly been about your failures. You ate too much yesterday. You were doomed and told yourself that you would eat too much that day. Or maybe you just woke up and ate whatever then regretted it afterward. Regardless, you were basically setting yourself and your day up for failure right from the start of it. Your first thought was negative so whatever happened next, like the first action you took, no matter what it was, was destined to be negative and the results had no other choice but to be negative. This isn't rocket science, right?

Remind yourself of one thing and remind yourself of it often. What I'm asking you to do is something that will *guarantee* you a good start to every single day. If your first thought is a positive one like being grateful for something, then your next action will match that gratitude and the result will be a positive one. What you do after that is up to you but I'm going to suggest more gratitude. It isn't hard to find things to be grateful for is it? When you're in your bathroom, is there toilet paper? Be grateful for it. Towels? Say thanks for the towels. Who cares what or whom you're thanking just be happy that you have them because if you are thinking positive thoughts, there is no room for you to be thinking negative thoughts.

There is a bunch of scientific data to back that theory but I'll keep it really simple. We are not designed to be both positive and negative at the same time. It's that simple. If we are feeding our minds positivity, it will crave more positivity and therefore, direct you toward finding more positivity. Be warned though, we are all living proof that the exact opposite is true as well and feeding our minds negativity will only create more opportunities to have negative results.

PLEASE READ: *There is an entire school of thought on this particular subject and if you want to learn more about it, I suggest strongly that you hop online and search for "The Secret" and "Law of Attraction" and Rhonda Byrne. I did those things and it changed my life in such a profound way that I am committed to paying it forward and passing along the knowledge any way that I can.*

Now, this next part is for those of you islands out there who are thinking that *you're the exception* and that you *can* be both positive and negative at the same time; which I promise you, you can't. It is absolutely impossible to think both positive thoughts and negative thoughts at the same time. I get it. You may think that you can *feel* positive and negative at the same time or maybe be happy and sad at the same time. No matter what though, one is always going to dominate and I'm going to be point-blank honest and tell you that if you think you can be both positive and negative at the same time you're absolutely wrong.

None of us are so unique that this concept is not 100% at work for us at all times. Regardless of which one you *choose,* you are always living your life in alignment with just one of them. Who am I kidding, those of you who are telling yourselves that you *can* be negative and positive at the same time are quite frankly, still hanging on to negativity and hopelessness and are *choosing* to believe that you are "different." Telling yourself that you are "different" is just another way for you to set yourself up to fail. It's a choice to think positively. It's as much of a choice to think negatively and the mere thought that you are convincing yourself that you are so different from everyone else is the exact same line or reasoning that you used to justify every mouthful of food that got you to a place of hopelessness to begin with. So if you are truly going to hang on to the idea that you are so different (and hopeless) that you actually can be grateful and ungrateful or happy and sad all at the same time, then my suggestion to you is to stop reading this book and go right back to doing the same things that you always did. Once you do, your misery and unhappiness and hopelessness will be refunded to you in full.

Keep something in mind though. If you choose to change your thinking right now, happiness and joy are also waiting for you. It's your choice. So if you're determined to be terminally unique, fine. Go ahead and keep right on believing that you can be negative and positive at the same time. It's your choice. It's a negative one though so stop lying to yourself and telling yourself otherwise. If you don't believe it's a choice, maybe you should go out and do a little more research. Maybe go so far as using the concept of gratitude against yourself by rushing to your favorite biggie-size spot and ordering up an unhealthy dose of despair to prove just how "different" you really are. Then try to tell yourself how grateful you are that you're different than the rest of us by convincing yourself that you're happy being fat, unhealthy and hopeless. The rest of us will be right here, seeing through our own BS and accepting that we share a common malady; we chose to be miserable and blamed food (and whatever else we could) for why we were so hopeless (i.e., negative) and would try anything to stop doing it, including being accepting that at least trying to be grateful is better than actively pursuing being ungrateful and subsequently unhappy.

Another option is that you can pause and think about it all and maybe take an honest assessment of yourself and at least try to stop being negative by not being so adamant about declaring your uniqueness about at the least, this particular aspect of your life. You can choose to at least try to be grateful for something without having to tie anything horrifying and negative to it just to prove that you're right and that me and a million other people are wrong. Regardless, whatever you choose to do is now and always has been your choice.

~ The Cost of Negativity ~

As I'm writing this and I mean, literally as I am typing this sentence on this page of this section of this book, my mom, who has been making horrifyingly negative food and eating choices for the better part of her life, is texting me about this exact topic. Ironic? Not really. In all actuality, it is exactly what I needed. As I sat looking at the next empty page contemplating the possible results of what I am going to write next, I managed to interject a quick gratitude thought into the mix. Why? Because what I'm about to write has the potential to cause some people to feel some really hard things and before the end of this section, some of you (us) will probably be forced to accept some really tough feelings and maybe even cry. That is why the last section on gratitude is so important to have at least read before moving forward.

You see, for me, being grateful has become a way of life now and I am holding on to the hope that it will for you as well. I have found that no matter what, if I bring gratitude with me, I am empowered to move in the direction of positivity. I've come to see the truth and that is that my life is either moving away from positivity or toward it but no matter what, I am the one making the choice of which direction to head.

So as I started this section, my mom was texting me about her own weight "loss" (or lack there of it). This is her exact text (copied and pasted with her permission): "I was on Jenny [Craig] for a year. Cost me at least $6,000.and I lost 35 pounds. Nutrisystem. Cost me $5,000 and I lost 18 pounds. I suck."

Yeah, so…that about sums it up, right? Do any of you identify with my mom on how, literally, costly the endeavor of "losing weight" (i.e., making one negative choice after the other) really is? The key to what my mom wrote is, "I suck." You know why? She has *no* problem identifying (anymore) with the fact that her inability to lose weight is *not* Jenny Craig's fault nor is it Nutrisystem's fault. Trust me when I say that was not always the case with my mom though. Truthfully, I am grossly understating the facts.

My mom is a hard case. Her denial ran and still runs so deeply that today, as I write this, she is just realizing that spending thousands of dollars on a diet program will never, ever work for her because in her own words, she sucks [at it]. The "it" for my mom is being able to make positive choices. She just can't do it. Truth be told, her entire kitchen is jam packed with Nutrisystem food because she and my dad have both been trying to lose "some" weight since the summer. It's now January. My dad, who thankfully will never read this, is a diabetic who is carrying at least 50 extra pounds around every day. My mom, two-time breast cancer SURVIVOR, is over 100 pounds overweight. Talk about ironic, right?

She's been on a "diet" for a lot of years now and at a current approximate expense of, as of today anyway, at least $11,000 and that is not including the money she has spent on other programs (aside from Jenny Craig and Nutrisystem) like Weight Watchers and The Atkins and South Beach diets. Also, that estimate does not include the thousands of dollars she's spent on diet books and paraphernalia like food scales or pedometers, etc. All of those are diet related things that she eventually used against herself to actually make sure that she was never, ever successful at the one thing that she wants more than anything in the world; to lose weight and be healthy.

I cannot tell you how many times I have heard her say, "There must be something wrong with my scale." Two months ago she actually went through the process of looking in the weekend's newspaper sale ads for scales that were on sale. Wow, how I identified with *that* particular line of negative reasoning. She has been on Nutrisystem for about a year now and has lost and gained the same 7 or 8 pounds on and off the entire time. She adds the losses up to come up with a cumulative total but she has never lost a significant enough amount to justify the cost, not that any of the technical diet things really matters when it comes right down to it.

The only thing that really matters is that there is a single, yes, one little thing, that she (and all of you, and I) refuses (refused, in some of our cases) to do. Change. It's that simple. It is one of the most important components needed to lose weight and it is universal to all of us. No matter what your health situation is like. No matter how much weight you have to lose and no matter what else you can think of that has to do with being overweight, obese, and fat or whatever else you want to call it. Without change, things stay the same. Diet after diet and attempt after attempt, without changing, you are nothing more than a hamster in a wheel chasing an end that doesn't exist.

The only thing in the way of my mother being able to lose weight is her own thoughts. Just because she admits to "sucking at" [losing weight] does not mean that she will miraculously start to lose any weight. Just because she accepts that it's her own fault doesn't mean that she has done anything to change the situation. Sucking at something implies negativity. It's a negative thought that will absolutely lead to a next negative action and that action with guarantee negative results.

It really is that simple. Does any of it sound familiar to any of you? It sure sounds spot on for me. Remember? I'm the one who blamed my scale for my own obesity and hopelessness and did so to the point of actually destroying it. You know what though, let me pause briefly to interject a much needed thought. In many cases, we all have at one time or another been so mad at food for *making us* fat and unhappy that we threw some of it away; uneaten. Let's keep it real though, how many of us regretted it at some point later and dug into the garbage and retrieved the food we had tossed out and then ate it? How many of us *honestly* took it out on the food itself? As if the food actually did something to us so heinous that we punished it by throwing it away.

I'm only bringing this up because this part of the book is about how much it cost us to live, no seek and maintain, a lifestyle of food indulgences and negativity. When it comes right down to it, buying food then getting mad at that food, then throwing it away and garbage picking it and maybe eating it or maybe throwing it away again or maybe trips to the drive thru and over eating then throwing up and buying books on diet and exercise or getting gym memberships and gym clothes and a gym bag or worse yet, buying treadmills and steppers and other at-home gym equipment that we all know gets used like twice then made into indoor clothes lines or conversation pieces…(deep breath)…oh, let's not forget the juicers. Oh God, the hundreds of dollars wasted on those nearly useless kitchen appliances. What about blenders and hundreds of dollars wasted on "healthy" foods that go totally rotten in the bottom drawer of the fridge or cupboard but that we hang on to until the last possible second as if *they* are our salvation because as long as they are there *they* somehow represent hope. Let's not ever forget the scales we tossed or blamed.

Honestly, I could go on and on and on (and on) and I bet you all have a few stories of your own that you could tell on the depths of the cost of the choices you made to maintain a life of absolute food related negativity. Just think about this though, with one thought of gratitude, you can be triggering an entire new destiny of inexpensive and sincere food related positivity. Why? Try it and you'll see for yourself, but I can tell you that not only is positivity good for your soul, it's good for your wallet as well. Think about how much it *really* cost to be obese and unhealthy?

Along with spending thousands of dollars on weight loss paraphernalia, let's touch on the literal cost of maintaining the body that houses that negative lifestyle you've chosen. Sure, most of us put our health last, especially when it comes to the foods we eat. None of us wants to be accountable for the physical toll that eating super-sized foods and drinks takes on our bodies but for the sake of this part of the book, we have to at least glance at it. I'll make it simple: Gall bladder disease. Kidney disease. Diabetes. Heart disease. Cellulitis. Cancer. Skin quality/rashes (essentially, food related allergies). Stomach and esophageal diseases along with a long list of chronic conditions related to those things. Should I keep going or can you identify with any of those? I sure could and still can, to be honest. My mom and dad, the only family I have, almost tap out the entire list right now. That's a sad reality check.

What? You don't think Tums and antacids count as part of the cost of maintaining a negative eating lifestyle? Really? Let me hit you with a little more reality. We'll call this my lead into the next chapter. I used to eat Tums like skittles. That went without saying since I ate skittles like skittles too. My gall bladder and stomach were so messed up that eating Tums was more normal for me than breathing. Then I changed my thinking and added some gratitude into my thoughts. Before long, my choices about what I ate started to change. Then my entire life started to change but before I even witnessed the miracle of positivity for myself, somewhere along the line (and I have no idea when), I stopped eating Tums like skittles; actually, I stopped eating skittles like skittles too. Actually, I stopped having to use Tums at all. Well, let me be honest, "at all" is relative to the bigger picture. . .and that leads us right straight to the next chapter.

CHAPTER 4
I Can't Weight!

I consider myself a RECOVERED negativity addict. I know those words sound harsh but "addict" can mean a lot of different things and the truth of the matter is that I really was addicted to it. All I ever wanted was more _____ (of whatever my current food obsession was). My thoughts were all about getting more and it didn't matter what the more was. It could have been McDonald's or skittles or stomachaches or low blood sugar or _____. I just wanted more of what I was already used to. No matter what, more for me always meant more of feeling awful and like a victim. Therefore, I got exactly what I asked for. My dominant thoughts were all and had been for a really long time, negative and all revolved around continuing to be a failure and hopeless and unhealthy, blah, blah, blah. The negative outweighed the positive (grossly understated). It's simple. My thoughts were poisoned with negativity and sadly I am the one who poisoned them (and myself).

I have to be honest and say that I was (will always) (on some level) be "addicted" to food (the kind of food that no one should ever eat the way I and we all have and still do). I was also addicted to everything that came with being a total junk food junkie, like the negative thoughts and actions and results. Ok. So there, I said it. Now you know. Does it change anything? It's a word and just because the world-at-large assigns negativity to it (addicted), I'm going to tell you that I choose not to sign on to the proverbial world-at-large and the negativity they have created around the word itself. Yes, being addicted is totally negative but admitting to being addicted is totally not negative. It's acceptance and it's a word so I simply accept it and move on from it. Using the word addicted is like having a bad cut on my finger and standing over it contemplating how bad it hurts and then asking myself whether and when I'll bleed to death all while I nearly bleed to death. Wouldn't it be better (and more positive) to accept that I'm cut and focus on stopping the bleeding and bandaging the thing up instead of wallowing in all of the worst-case scenarios about the thing? You all know exactly what I'm talking about, too. Acceptance is the cut (or being addicted to food). It happened. I chose not to allow it to make me bleed to death and accepted it and fixed it.

All I'm saying is that your weight and eating habits and hopelessness and despair, etc. are all now and have always been nothing more and nothing less than the result of the choices that you made. Choices that started as thoughts then led to actions and those actions ended in results and there is no gray area here. It's all about two things: positivity or negativity. Each needs the other to survive but neither cares a thing about the other. Don't give me some line of BS about batteries and other things that use the two simultaneously either because for the most part, you'll just be making my point for me (and kind of making a total ass out of yourself). My point? Either you're headed toward positivity or away from it. If you need scientific proof, lick a battery.

This entire book is about helping you move from where you are now to a place where you have always wanted to be. Whether you fully accept it yet or not, you can't wait to change your weight. Sure, you mind may be playing tricks on you and telling you to stop reading this book. That's what your mind has done with every other diet related thing that you have ever done up until this point. Regardless of what you choose to do, what you have read in *this* book will change you whether you want it to or not. I've worked with a lot of people just like you. Scared. Reluctant. Skeptical. Angry. Resentful. You name it and I have had a client who has felt it. The main thing you need to know about my program and tools is that they *will* work for you no matter what you think. My program isn't a thinking program. It's an action program.

CHAPTER SKINNY
It's Just a Word

This book is not (and I never intended it to be) something righteous and coming at you from some pious point of view as if I am the all seeing and all knowing on this particular subject. Truth-be-told, in the time that it has taken me to write this book I've gone from a person who eats 100% "clean" or "healthy" and in alignment with what is considered "positive" eating to a person who falters, like the imperfect person who I admittedly am. I have absolutely eaten "negatively" since I first started my own weight loss (and acceptance) journey. Hey, it's all about being honest (with myself), right?

The thing is, *what* I've eaten is not as important as the fact that I *have*, at this point of my life, a heightened awareness of the depths that negativity can and will take me *if I let it*. For me, every day is about the same thing; moving *more* in the direction of positivity than heading non-stop, hopelessly into the darkness and direction of negativity. I still make poor choices and by poor choices I mean, negative ones. I also pay the price for them because there is one thing I can attest to with conclusive and unfaltering evidence; that a single negative thought, will and always does end with a negative action and that action, will, with absolute precise accuracy, end in a negative result. No matter how big or small the thought, the action and result will fall in line with it.

For example: One unstopped thought about a bag of Cheetos ends in the purchase of a bag of Cheetos, which ends in eating that bag of Cheetos, which in turn (we all know this ends with an empty bag of Cheetos, right?). . .and so the negativity train is well on its way to Negative Ville. You know what I mean, don't you? How many times have you all said something about starting over tomorrow? Or how many of you have gone to bed holding you stomachs from overeating? How many trips have you made for Tums because of the choices you've made; choices to allow one little bit of negativity back into you thoughts?

I need you all to notice something really important though ok? I said "one *unstopped* thought about [a bag of Cheetos] . . ." because there is a caveat to the whole gratitude/positive/negative thing. Most of us ended up in an overall hopeless state of food related negativity because no one ever told us that we could change our thoughts *at any time*. Yes, you read that right. We need to be told or given permission to be imperfect and to make mistakes. It seems so simple, just like the gratitude thing, but really, it isn't. Most of us hold ourselves to some unobtainable level of perfection as if we are Gods, but let me tell you right here and now, we're not Gods. Further, being non-stop positive means we would be non-stop perfect and none of us, NONE of us are perfect!

One of the primary goals of this book is to get you to understand how important it actually is to change your thinking (right now, this very second) so that there is an immediate shift in your thought patterns. In other words, by the time you are done reading this book, you want to make it so that positivity outweighs (pun intended) negativity and not just in your thoughts. This is a change in your thoughts that will trigger a cause and effect that is life changing. I am talking about thoughts that lead to an immediate action. They are also thoughts that can and will change all of your future actions and subsequently, the results of your entire life. I know. You're thinking that by this point in the book you were expecting *me* to have done something to actually cure you. I'm sorry, but I'm not a miracle worker. This one's on you. All I can do is give you the tools that you need to succeed and I am so willing to do that. Like I said in an earlier chapter though, if *you* use them, *your* success is guaranteed. My part is to coach you along the way and give you the tools that you need to succeed. Keep in mind that if you choose not to use my help and tools, there's another guarantee. Without doing the work it takes to change your current eating habits and weight your misery and desperation *will* be refunded to you as well.

As your coach, at least up until this point anyway, I think you should keep pushing forward and at least try my program and tools out. I mean you have already read up until this point. You should at least give what I'm suggesting a shot. You can start by being grateful that I *can't* fix you. The end result is going to be an overwhelmingly positive feeling of self-respect and accomplishment and it will all be because of you! Then be grateful that everything that I just told you is proven to work. It hasn't just worked for me in my life. This will work for **anyone** who chooses to use it. It's even working for my mom, who for the most part hasn't lost a significant enough amount of weight for it to no longer be taking a financial or physical toll on her but I have watched her change her thoughts (almost in spite of herself). I have watched her go from a person who blamed everyone (including me) and everything (the scale, food, even her doctors) for her obesity and negativity to a person who at least sees through her own BS enough to see what *her* part in it is. And believe me, the scale blaming incident that she just went through is just one tiny step forward for her. A step forward is, not matter what, an action though. I just told you how my program is not a thinking program but an action program. That is a very important thing to remember. My mom is aware of the fact that she cannot think herself out of the situation that she is in. The thing is, it's *her* journey to *her* destiny and it is up to *her* when she'll arrive and how she'll get there. Just like it took me whatever it took for me to change my destiny and just like it's up to *you* when and how *you* <u>will</u> get to your new destiny.

It's all relative to our thoughts. I do understand that. Thoughts and actions go hand in hand. It's all relative to when the scales are tipped more toward positive thinking than they are toward negative thinking though. The laws of physics are not pliable; they are as fixed as the law of positivity (or negativity, if you so choose). We all have a different tipping point but no matter what, the law is the law and if we put more time and energy into one or the other, that is the one that will dictate our lives. A thought, actions, results. The choice is ours. Do we tip the scales to the positive or the negative? No matter what, no one or thing holds our destiny in their or its hands but ourselves.

We each choose which tools we are going to use and when and how we will use them. There is one thing that you can do to insure your own success though. It is to vigilantly believe in yourself every day, through gratitude. No matter what else you do, start being grateful and it doesn't even matter for what you are grateful or when. Just start being grateful and let gratitude do the work and block out the negative thoughts that will be trying to get through. Then before you know it, the positive will outweigh the negative and the rest will just sort of start to work itself out. If you remember how one positive thought will lead to one positive action and that will bring you one positive result then just start to imagine what multiplying that chain by a day's worth of positive thoughts can do. It's like you're building a chain mail suit of armor around yourself to help block out any negativity that tries to hurt (kill) you. Acceptance, gratitude, destiny.

You can start anytime you want. You can even start over anytime that you want. Even if you've been on a cycle of negativity, you have the power to stop it at anytime. Just accept your part in it and then accept that you made negative choices and got exactly what you asked for. Then be grateful for anything. Maybe be grateful for the opportunity to imperfectly try to tip the scales of your own thoughts toward working with you instead of against you again. Be grateful that you don't have to be perfect. Be grateful that now you know that your obesity and unhealthy state of being (physical and mental) had nothing to do with the biggie size meals but everything to do with your (negative) thoughts around them.

Start by being accepting of what is undeniable like the fact that there is little positive that comes from spending money or eating that biggie sized meal, but the truth is the truth and if you *choose* to pay for that meal and then eat it, there will be equal results to the choices that you made. For the sake of your own destiny, those choices are either bringing you closer to positivity or farther away from it. Whether you eat the biggie meal or not is irrelevant if you disregard the truth of the matter because otherwise, why even bother? Not thinking your (our) actions through is what got you (us) where you (we) were in the first place, right? This is why my three questions are so important.

~ Unzip the Fat Suit ~

I don't know about you, but back when I first laughed at my hopeless situation and myself and then accepted my part in it all, I decided to try, every single day, to take more steps toward Positivity Land than I had been taking to the Land of Gloom and Doom. I get it. There is more to it all. Right now it probably feels like you're zipped inside of a fat suit and that the zipper is stuck, but is it really stuck? We all want to be some ideal thing like "skinny" because we're tired of being this other thing, "fat" but those are just words, like "American" or "Italian" or "_____." You can't *be* something (skinny) unless you think about *it* more than you think about everything else. Just like you *are* the very thing that you spend the most time thinking about not being (fat). Get it? You can't just will the fat suit to unzip itself and fall off of you. Especially since you're the one who zipped yourself inside of it in the first place. The more you keep telling yourself the zipper is stuck, the longer it will stay stuck. Thoughts lead to actions, remember?

So what do you do to get out of the fat suit? Accept that you didn't end up in a fat suit by osmosis. Accept the truth; that *you zipped yourself inside of it* and then did everything that you could to stay there. Then decide that you want out and start using your new tools. Be grateful for the awareness of the fact that you put yourself exactly where you are. Then ask yourself if by being inside of the fat suit is causing you to walk toward positivity or away from it? Are you headed for a solution or have you packed a bag and decided to camp out in the problem? If you want out of the fat suit that you're in and you believe that the zipper is stuck, grab some scissors and start cutting yourself out of it. . .it's *your* destiny. Where it ends and begins (and maybe even ends and begins again) has always been, is now, and always will be. . .up to *you*.

The zipper is only stuck if you believe it is.

~~THE END~~
The Beginning

If you're (still) wondering where the chapter is where I tell you what to eat to lose weight you'll be looking for a long time. I never told you that this is a diet book. It isn't a recipe book and it isn't really a self-help book either. It's a how-to book. It's a book meant to teach you how to change the person who you have been into the person who you want to be and unfortunately, the only person who can *really* change you is you. If you really think about everything that you've read in the previous chapters, you probably had a strong feeling that there wouldn't be a section in the book where I coddle you and tell you exactly what to do next. I said it already and I'll say it again, acceptance is a vital tool that can and will change your life no matter what. It is (still) up to you how and when you use it though.

Besides, at this point, do you even believe that diets "work" or that me telling you which one to choose will make any more sense than me telling you to go to KFC and buy a biggie bucket for one with a side of gravy slathered potatoes? I'm not in control of you. You have to unzip yourself from the fat suit that you've trapped yourself inside of. As your coach, I can suggest that you use the tools that I've just told you about but that is as far as me telling you how, what or when to do anything will go. It really is time for you to accept responsibility for yourself and where you are with your eating habits and weight issues. I really mean it when I say I can't fix you for you.

Don't panic though. It doesn't mean I'm going to just leave you hanging. I'll at least give you as much insight and help along the way that I can. I know that this all is so much digest (pun intended, again). That's why at the end of the book I will direct you to my web site and even offer you personal coaching. I don't expect you feel like you are alone in this. I said that right from the start. At this point though, I do expect you to accept that you and only you can take the actions necessary to actually change yourself. Part of doing that is learning how to armor your new self in defense against the thoughts that had you trapped in the fat suit by your old self.

Now, as your coach, at least until the end of the book, I will start helping you discover ways to use your Life Success Tools to build a new suit of armor. One that you don't feel trapped in like that old fat suit that you wore for so many years. Let me start to help you defend yourself against ever having to go back to the old you by telling you what I've learned on the subject of diets.

~ Diets Decoded ~

As I am writing this book (and I mean yesterday, literally) my dad, the guy I told you is 50 pounds over weight and a diabetic, went to Barnes and Noble and bought one of Dr. Fuhrman's books on diabetes or eating to cure diabetes or some other diet related book. That is after he painstakingly looked online for *any* book about diabetes and how to cure it with a diet. So as my dad sits upstairs at the dining room table flipping through another diet book, I am downstairs writing a book about the same topic and the irony is, he's heard me talk. He's watched me change. I have helped both him and my mom by actually putting together individual eating plans for each of them that have worked for them both. I have coached them both and they know exactly what to do to have exactly what I have which is my health and significant weight loss. Sadly though, my dad in particular is almost adamant about *not* changing. He has approximately $700 worth of Nutrisystem food scattered on the kitchen table and counters (next to my mom's Nutrisystem food, of course). He knows how to eat on the Nutrisystem program and he also knows that he will lose weight on that program.

Let me back up just a little to really solidify my point. After my dad went to Barnes and Noble last night (to buy one of Dr. Fuhrman's diet books), he made a quick drive thru at Taco Bell and ordered up some gluttonous denial for himself and my mom. Then, book in hand, dad came home and spent a few hours eating Taco Bell then digging around the fridge and cabinets for chips or anything else he could get his hands on (other than the Nutrisystem food scattered all over his kitchen). Then, at some point later when I texted my mom to see what they were doing, she told me that my dad was reading the book and was really excited about it. She even quoted something from the book that said something about Fuhrman's plan being like gastric bypass without the surgery. What?! So without hesitation I texted this back, "You know what though, it's good that he's reading it but he doesn't have a good track record with acceptance..... He needs to read my book." and then I took a deep breath and texted this, "if he doesn't accept HIS part in his own diabetes and I mean really accept it, then he is destined to just keep reading books on how to fix it without ever really fixing it."

My parents are no different than most of us when it comes to diets. We've tried them all, mostly in desperate attempts of self-preservation but only after we hit another undeniable bottom. For years my mom would binge eat the worst foods possible and then run to that all protein fad diet. She would last a few weeks on that diet and then it was right back to the chocolate and denial diet. My dad, who is as proverbially literally addicted to soda and junk food as it gets (eating take out seven days a week and always buying it for my mom as well), has absolutely no self-control at all. He even pretended he didn't have diabetes until it got to the point where he was no longer able to ignore the physical effects of the disease. Well, that and his doctor put him on insulin for his out of control blood sugar levels. For my dad, acceptance for his diabetes came in the form of a pill bottle.

My parents are my hardest cases. They have proven to me over and over again a something that I had already learned the hard way myself. The lesson is that diets will never, ever, ever, EVER work for anyone who does not *first* accept their part in why they even need the diet in the first place. My dad, like so many other people, is reading another diet book hoping that a cure miraculously pops off of one of the pages and magically absorbs into his system leaving him instantaneously cured of his obesity, diabetes, denial, addiction, obsession, etc., etc. He has absolutely no plan to commit to the diet in Dr. Fuhrman's book. Well, he'll commit to it for about a week or maybe two. He'll lose some weight and start feeling better and then he'll forget that he ever felt horrible in the first place. Then, on the first day that he *really* feels good, he will think that the book cured him and he will celebrate by taking himself our for a congratulatory round of super sized take out. The next morning, he will have guilt, remorse and shame over how ill the celebratory eating binge felt from the night before. His blood sugar will be out of control again, he'll gain back the weight he lost and alas, the hamster is back inside of the wheel.

It isn't the good doctor's diet's fault for why my dad will fail (again). It's my dad's fault. Believe me, I am no hypocrite. I did the exact same thing that my dad is doing and tried every single diet out there, even the same ones that my parents are still trying. I really do mean almost every diet out there. I even went a few steps beyond what most people I know have done to try to lose weight and tried life threatening diet pills. I am talking about the diet pills that actually ended up killing people. I also tried all shake diets and all grapefruit diets. I tried detox diets and soup diets. You get he picture, right?

Now that you know that I am just like the rest of you except with a few years of successful use of my own program and tools to call upon to help you, I am going to solidify a very important point. I will say this again and again and again until you get sick of hearing it but it's something that is very important to understand: Diets do not work unless the person dieting has committed to *making* them work. At this point I could tell you all the name of the diet that finally "worked" for me but it is a moot point. The diet had nothing to do me finally succeeding and losing a bunch of weight. I am the one who did the work. I am the one who accepted that the reason why diets never worked for me before was because a diet and food are inanimate objects and have no power over me at all. I am the one who gave up fighting and blaming and obsessing and denying and took 100% accountability for my own destiny. Hell, it's a diet, not a miracle cure in a book, bottle or box. I'm the one who got myself into the fat suit. I had to be the one to get myself out and it wasn't easy, believe me but I am so grateful for where I am today. I am even more grateful to be able to share how I got here with you.

The next thing that I am going to tell you about diets is something that actually saved my life. It did so by making it so that I could no longer blame *them* for all of my failed attempts at dieting. Because of what I just said in the last paragraph, I gained a solid understanding of just how much diets do not participate in the actual act of weight lose (or gain). Through my own acceptance of what diets are *not*, I was forced to finally understand what exactly they *are*.

Diets are nothing more and nothing less than a *set of directions* on how to lose weight. They are as literally as you can take them, nothing more than instructions on how to eat stuff that will help your body go into a mode of losing weight. You're probably think something like 'There, she summed up what a diet really is. Now I can go off on my own and lose a bunch of weight.' Hang on though. Before you go rushing off with that information, let me put it a little clearer for you. Although diets are instructions on how to lose weight, they *still* don't work without *you* following the directions.

Imagine that you just bought one of those desks in a box and when you get it home, you need to unpack the pieces and assemble the desk. What do you do first? Most people who are building something like that will unpack all of the pieces then grab the instructions and read them to see what tools they need to assemble the thing, right? Most people don't just dump the pieces on the floor and then go to sleep, expecting the pieces to put themselves together so when they wake up the thing is all together and set up. That sounds absolutely crazy doesn't it?

45

So keeping that scenario in mind, think about the next diet that you are going to try as nothing more than a set of instructions on how to lose weight. First you pick the diet. Then you read the instructions and get to work putting the thing together. I already loaded your toolbox with some of the tools that you need. It's up to you to follow the diet's instructions and then build the body (and life) that you want. Trust me, I know how you feel right now. This is probably a really scary thought. At this point, you have to accept the reality that diets actually *do* work. Then you have to accept that it *really* was you who was to blame for *all* of the prior failed attempts that you made at losing weight.

I promise you, I really do know how overwhelming it can feel right now. I am the one who looked at my old destiny and accepted that the food and diets that I spent years blaming for my own pathetic failures had nothing to do with my obesity and failing health. I am the one who stopped believing that the scale was conspiring against me and I am the one who made a conscious choice to change the person who I was and believe me when I tell you, it was not easy at all. It was however, worth every single second of acceptance and growth that it took for me to get to the other side of that old destiny and to this place where my new destiny exists. And it all started with laughter and a single positive, acceptance based thought where there was no longer any way that I could deny accountability. Diets do work. Ok? They are instructions and that is all. Got it? So throw away your old ideas about them and just move on. Acceptance, remember?

~ Instructions and Tools ~
* **Believe** *

At this point, I'm going to give you something else that I know that you have been waiting for. I waited until the end of the book to give this to you because I want it to be something that you keep fresh in your minds as you close the book and venture out on your own journeys. Before I give it to you though, I need to remind you of something:

Positive thoughts lead to positive actions that lead to positive results. The opposite is absolutely and completely the case and *negative thoughts lead to negative actions that lead to negative results.* Always remember that. Repeat it often. Write it down somewhere if you need to but always keep it close.

Ok, so now I can give you the final tool for your success toolbox. If you start a diet and **believe** that you will succeed, you *will* succeed. There. That's it. The final tool is simple but powerful and it is as easy as this: believe in yourself. The *only* reason diets have never worked for you in the past is because you started them with negativity and disbelief. You were more than likely, just like my dad, looking for a quick and easy way out of a bad situation but had no intention of actually doing anything differently than you had been doing. Either you were feeling sick or knew that it was unhealthy to gain so much weight in such a short period of time or just didn't like your clothes not fitting anymore or whatever your reasons were. Time and time again though, you failed and it was always because you told yourself that you would fail.

Sure, some of you will say that you started strong and don't know what happened but you still ended up quitting the diet. Others will say that they lost momentum and had every intention of making the diet work but got bored or _____ (fill in the blank with whatever excuse you used). Some of you will even say that you had what you call total success and lost all the weight that you wanted to and then gained the weight back (usually plus a bunch more) and have no idea what happened. I've seriously heard it (or lived it personally) all when it comes to this topic. Trust me when I tell you that had you ever truly accepted things for what they actually were and then became grateful for everything and anything and then realized that *you* were the one in control of your own destiny (i.e., the one to blame), then the believing in yourself part would have happened in spite of you and you would have lost the weight and kept it off and would never be reading this book.

Truthfully, there are times when I don't believe that my mom actually wants to lose weight. She is homebound at this point because of her obesity and can hardly get around anymore. She blames it on this thing or that and her most recent excuse is her knees being "bad" which they absolutely are. She's 4'11" and weighs just shy of 300 pounds. Of course her knees are bad. Those knees are her most recent excuse though and are just the end of a long list of other excuses she's used over the years. Sadly, my mom is such a happy and grateful person that it's super hard to see her still hanging on to her old destiny. She's even one of those people who you would think could be both positive and negative at the same time. You know, the people I wrote about in the chapter about gratitude. The islands who believe that they are terminally unique and that there is no help *for* them.

Yes, that's my mom. She has even said that she is a hopeless case and that she doesn't believe that she is able to lose weight. It's her knees or her thyroid or her DNA or her genes or she is weak or whatever other thing that she can cling onto that is *outside of herself*. In other words, she believes that her destiny is not something that she can control. So she has just given up on everything to do with weight loss. She's apathetic and miserable and desperate and hopeless all at the same time yet she believes that she is grateful too and she actually is. Here's the clincher though. She, like the rest of us, cannot be both positive and negative at the same time.

What I'm saying is that she spends *more* time focusing on being a failure than she does on being a success. Believing in her failures is still believing in herself though. It's just that believing that she's a failure tips the scales more toward negativity than positivity so subsequently, her life and destiny are headed non-stop and one-way toward full on negativity. Although she appears to be grateful and happy, she never has fully accepted her part in her own destiny, the destiny of food obsession and obesity that will more than likely kill her. The saddest thing about that is that even if she just accepts herself as an obese woman who likes to eat really unhealthy foods, she is by default, tipping the scales a tiny bit toward positivity. That one thought really may just be enough to start moving her toward the true acceptance and gratitude that she needs to start tipping the scales more toward positivity.

That's where *my* acceptance has to come in though. She is my mom and I want so badly to see her succeed like I have. The truth of the matter is that whenever I work with anyone who believes they are struggling and refuses to change, my heart aches a lot for them. I know how they feel. I know where they are but I also know that I too was hopeless and desperate and even tried to kill myself because I really didn't believe there was a way out. My dad, deeply involving himself inside of another diet book, will absolutely not lose any weight. His diabetes will not be cured, no matter what Dr. Fuhrman's books tells him and none of you will miraculously wake up tomorrow skinny. No matter how much I wish I *could* wave a magic wand and have that happen for each and every one of you, I can't and it won't. You, like my parents, have to want to save yourselves and the only way to do it is to find your instructions, pick up your tools and start building the life that you want. It's your story and your destiny, not mine.

When I told you that we all have a story, I meant it literally. This is where it will all make more sense. Part of acceptance of this entire topic is that some people's stories end filled with the same negativity that they began with. You see, if you hang on to negativity, the outcome *will* be more and more opportunities to be negative and that means right up to death. Some people will actually and literally die trying - trying *to* change or trying *not to* change. If a person believes that they cannot lose weight then everything that they do and become will align them with situations where they have opportunity after opportunity to *not* lose weight. The good news is that if any person believes that they can and will lose weight, then everything that they do and become will align them with opportunities for them to lose weight. We all create the destiny that we want. We write our own story.

It is 100% up to you what happens next. It doesn't matter which diet you choose or whether you try one and then ditch it and then try another. You can even choose not to diet and to stay exactly how you are except for the part where you start to accept the things that you did that made you feel hopeless and desperate. It's your destiny. Remember that. Also remember that whatever you choose to do from this very point on, your life is completely and absolutely up to you. I don't just mean the choices that you make either. I mean the outcomes as well.

Take some time to think back over your life and think about a time when you wanted to lose weight but believed something like the odds were against you. Then really assess the entire situation. Ask yourself the hard questions and really accept everything for exactly what it was. Did you believe that you would lose weight? Ever? Did you do things to guarantee your success or did you spend more time and energy making sure you failed? Every single time that you tried to lose weight, you were in total control of the outcome.

The law of gratitude and the law of acceptance and the law of destiny are all impersonal. They will work no matter what and no matter where and no matter when you call upon them. They don't even care whether you succeed or fail. They exist like the law of gravity. What goes up will come down, you know? If you're grateful for where you've been and accept it and then choose to change the things about yourself that you don't really like or need anymore, like magic, you will achieve exactly what you ask for. Be positive, the result will [always] be positive. Be negative and don't stop the negativity and the result will [always] be negative. You get what you ask for.

If looking back over the times that you tried to lose weight doesn't prove to you that you were more negative than positive and that is why you failed, then test what I am saying in your current life. Go out and try it on something little. Try telling yourself that you want to eat something "bad" and then accept it for what it is or accept it for what it isn't. Ask yourself the three questions that I told you about in Chapter 2. Think it through and assess it and accept it. Then realize that you can be grateful that you have the choice and finally, be prepared to own the affect it has on the destiny you are headed for (no matter what you choose).

If eating an entire pizza by yourself will fit into your new destiny, go for it. Even if it won't fit into that new destiny and you go for it anyway, you still have the tools and can use them at *any time* and they *will* still work. All you have to do if you choose to eat something that doesn't make you feel good about yourself is accept it for what it really is. Accept that you ate it and that you probably didn't really want or need to eat it and that there are repercussions from the choice you made, then move on. Don't dwell in the negativity. Don't let one incident own your destiny and especially do not ever go backward and move more toward negativity than positivity. Tell yourself repeatedly that diets *do* work and that they are just instructions. Then tell yourself that sometimes you put something together wrong and have to take it apart and build it again. Telling yourself those things will keep you moving in a positive direction instead of telling yourself that you are a failure because you made one mistake.

If you haven't figured it out yet, what I'm telling you is that this is a process. It's not a cure or quick fix. Your new destiny is a journey of trial and error but it does come with instructions and it also comes with tools. When you finish reading this book, I suggest that you choose any diet that feels right to you and then believe in yourself right form the beginning (even if it is half heartedly). Tell yourself over and over that you will succeed as long as you follow the instructions and use the tools that you've been given. Be grateful for every little thing that you can along the way. Accept that you are where you are because of your own choices but that you can make new choices and yes, you really can create a new destiny. Tell yourself that whichever diet you choose can and will work for you. Tell yourself that over and over again because if you are telling yourself that, then you are *not* telling yourself the opposite; that basically no matter which diet you chose, *it* won't work.

Understand? And don't be afraid to falter and I beg you, don't try to do it perfectly. Just keep accepting and being grateful and believing in yourself and try to visualize a new destiny and you really will start to change. The hopelessness will start to disappear. You will no longer feel desperate and controlled by food and make poor choices because you will innately begin to make really great choices; life changing choices and it will feel like it is happening in spite of yourself. Losing weight will stop being something horrifying and scary and villainous because you will have accepted that it has no control over you anymore. Food will stop being animated and lifelike and you will see it for what it really is, food.

Remember something though, at any time that you choose, you will be returned to the old, negative person who you were if you start making choices to do so. So don't ever let your guard down. Please, no matter what happens, find gratitude in anything that you can. It's a go-to tool and will save you when you think that things are starting to feel bad again. Be honest with yourself though. Tell yourself that things *will* feel bad sometimes because no one is perfect and part of the journey is testing the path for stability. There will be times when you doubt the positivity and will step into a puddle only to find out that it is really quicksand. It will only be after you fight your way out of that quicksand that you will realize that you should have just played it safe and walked around that mud puddle in the first place. Trial and error though, right? Sometimes you will make a choice that feels like a set back but if you're grateful for it and accept it, you will see that you have learned what *not* to do (again) in the future. Sometimes it's just as important to learn what you don't want as it is to know what you do want.

I can tell you all that I vehemently do not want to be like my parents (anymore). I love them dearly but where they are is not where I want to be anymore. I walked down the roads they are walking and fell in the quicksand over and over and I am grateful for having done so but going back is just not an option anymore. They teach me, on a daily basis, what I don't want to do and sadly, that is one of those acceptances that are tough but necessary. I have my own instructions and so do they. Sure, I still try to help and coach them but I do it from a safe distance because truth be told, if I go to Taco Bell with them, I will not be ordering a salad. You know what I'm saying? It is so easy to give in and I have and every time I do, I have to ask myself the same questions that I've told you to ask. I've indulged and overeaten with them and even last night, when my dad was going to Taco Bell for himself and mom, they asked if I wanted anything and I said no.

So you see, I am faced with the hard questions every day and I do give in sometimes but so far, I just shake it off and pick up the pieces and start over at the next meal and I'm a better person for it. I let positivity dominate my thoughts no matter what. I live in gratitude and I mean real gratitude. I have even sat holding my stomach saying how grateful I am for the stomachache (from over eating) because being grateful helps me fully accept responsibility for it and defuses any chances of me lying to myself and blaming the food or my parents or _____. The result of me personally utilizing the tools that I've told you all about is that I've lost a lot of weight (a lot) and have kept it off. I've done so even with having my little bouts of making bad choices because no matter what, I stay positive, try to enjoy the food no matter what and own the result (which often is a stomach ache and regret). I just don't pack a bag and live in the negativity and allow myself to quit completely.

I don't have gal bladder or kidney or liver problems anymore and my blood sugar rarely goes low anymore. I'm happier than I have ever been in my entire life and I accept something today that I was always afraid and ashamed to accept before. I love food but I hated being fat. I mean it when I say that I really love food too. I am no longer afraid or ashamed to admit it either. I just don't let that love dictate the relationship anymore. Part of that comes from accepting the reality of being fat and uncomfortable and really having to accept how much I hated the fact that I made myself those things.

So as I close this book out, I'm simply going to tell you that I believe in you and I hope that you start to believe in yourself as well. It may seem hard at first but as long as you don't let negativity dominate your thoughts and actions and results, you can and will live a life beyond your wildest imagination. Just practice giving yourself permission to falter and to be imperfect but remember when you don't get it perfect that it is not the end of the journey for you. It's just an opportunity to pick up a tool and fix something that isn't working. It really is simple. If you head toward negativity, you will just get more and more opportunities to live a life filled with negativity but if you head more toward positivity, you really will be given more opportunities to live a life filled with more and more positivity.

Don't set out to get it perfect though. Believing in yourself means doing so *unconditionally* and no matter what happens. So even if you have a "bad meal" or even a "bad day" don't let your belief falter. Do not let a bad day turn into a bad week or month or year or life. Use your instructions and tools. Tell yourself over and over that you can restart a diet or a day over at any time. If you eat something horrible for lunch, pick yourself up and get back on track for dinner. If you choose to take a day off from eating on whichever diet you choose, fine, commit to it then accept it then stay positive about it. Do not let negativity tell you that since you had one day off of your diet or meal plan that it won't matter it you have another day off. When one day off turns into another then another *those* are the exact negative thoughts that perpetuated and got you to that non-stop, one-way ride to hopelessness and despair in the first place. Always keep that in the front of your mind. Accept it and own it and be accountable for it.

Those are probably among some of the most important things that I can tell you because I've been there and I have fallen apart and I promise you, once I allowed myself to become negative again, my misery and despair and hopelessness were refunded to me ten times quicker and worse than you can possibly ever imagine. So when I tell you that it is easier to stay on the path to positivity than it is to get back on it after falling off, I hope more than anything in this world, you believe me and take my advice because back then, I sure wasn't using it. The tools work. You just have to pick them up and start using them, even if it feels awkward at first. What I'm saying is just keep plowing forward *no matter what* because from right now on, you SO got this!!!

You don't have to die trying. You can live succeeding!
  Your journey to the most amazing destiny ever begins right NOW. . .

Success is only a thought away!

~ NOTES ~

<u>Life Success Tools</u>

Acceptance (pg. 20)

_____

_____

_____

_____

_____

_____

_____

_____

Destiny (pg. 21)

_____

_____

_____

_____

_____

_____

_____

_____

Gratitude (pg. 25)

_____

_____

_____

_____

_____

_____

_____

_____

Believe (pg. 47)

_____

_____

_____

_____

_____

_____

_____

_____

_____

_____

_____

~ Three Questions ~
(pg. 14)

_____

_____

_____

_____

_____

_____

_____

_____

_____

_____

_____

_____

_____

_____

_____

_____

_____

_____

_____

_____

_____

_____

Annette Blake

<u>Weight Loss Consultant and Coach</u>

Annette Blake has over 10 years experience working as a
Weight Loss Consultant & Coach. She has worked extensively
on a 1-on-1 basis with clients but has also worked for a major
weight loss company. Her experience has enabled her to obtain
a solid understanding of the world of weight loss consulting
and coaching.

As a person who has been on her own weight loss journey
(most of her life) and finally achieved absolute success and
freedom from her own seemingly desperate and hopeless
weight gain, she is very compassionate about helping others do
the same. Being compassionate is not enough for Annette
though. She is also committed and extremely passionate about
helping people not just lose weight, but in helping them
decode the "mystery" behind why the diets they repeatedly try
have not "worked" so that they never have to make the same
mistakes of weight loss followed by weight gain again.

In her newest book, The Fat [Skinny] American; Book One:
Diets Decoded, Annette proves just how committed she is to
helping others by not only telling her own story, but offering a
set of Life Success Tools that she used and still uses today and
is so confident that they can and will work for <u>anyone who
uses them</u> that she guarantees their success.

Life Coach

Along with working as a weight loss consultant, Annette has also worked as a life coach and has helped people in all aspects of their lives. Some of her coaching has included post-weight loss transitioning. Although Annette's main focus is weight loss consulting and coaching, she has also coached many people and helped them focus on building a life beyond their wildest imagination.

Author

Annette *the author* has published a wide variety of books including adult romantic comedies and young adult fiction. She has also written poetry, essays, screenplays, theater pieces and plays and has worked as a freelance reporter for a large newspaper. She is also an accomplished blogger and has a very popular blog of which she has managed and maintained since 2010.